ELENA SHOSHITAISHVILI

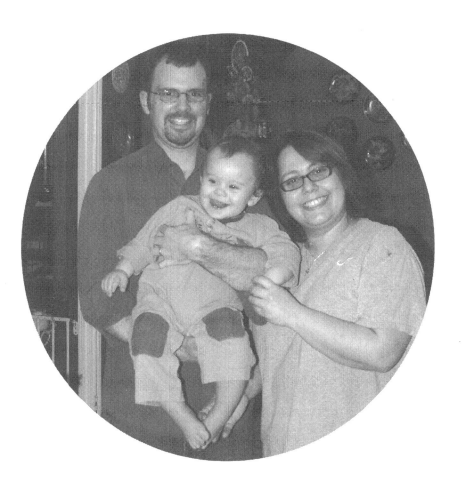

CHEMO SAGA

"My husband shaved my head"
and other great stories.

Disclaimer:

Although all stories in this Saga are true, the author could be suffering from bouts of slight exaggeration at times. I blame it on the drugs!

Acknowledgements:

I would like to thank my family, especially my husband Richard, for providing endless support and a rich and wonderful source of material for my Saga.

Other books by the same author:

Geophysical investigation of Archean and Proterozoic crustal-scale boundaries in Wyoming and Colorado with emphasis on the Cheyenne Belt.

Photo on previous page: Our family two days after my first chemo treatment

Prolog

February 18, 2008

Dear Family and Friends,

It seems that lots of things have happened to me in the last month and a half.

It all started when I found a lump on the bottom of my neck coming back from Christmas vacation. Since then I have had a whole bunch of scans and tests and been prodded in a whole bunch of places and aspirated and surgically removed and so on... As a result of it all I have a proof that I have a brain that is bigger then a walnut, but unfortunately there is no proof that it is functional and the report said that it is rather unremarkable... Not something you want to put on your resume...

However, I also have a diagnosis, which is that I have a lymphoma. Lymphoma is a type of cancer that originates in lymphocytes (a type of white blood cell in the vertebrate immune system). There are many types of lymphoma and most of them are manageable with a high success rate.

*From the letter asking to sponsor me in **Katy Relay for Life**.*

Chapter 1

February 15, 2008

O.k....

Here is the story of the last couple of days:

On Monday I had bone marrow test done. I was told by the doctor that I am the first patient that laughed on the table during the procedure. But imagine this: you lay on your stomach with your pants pulled down (the bone marrow extraction is from the hips). You are covered with a blanket from head to waist and from waist to toes. So the only thing that the doctor sees is your naked butt. And in order to take your attention away from the pain and other unpleasantness of the situation he chats with you...well really with your butt... about kids. So I started laughing.

On Tuesday I had a port installed. Well that was not a pleasant procedure! But the funny part was that they had to give me a double dose of the sedatives to relax me and I still kept talking! The washing blood out of my hair later at home was not very nice also, so overall I didn't like that whole procedure.

On Wednesday we went to get the first dose of chemo... that wasn't too bad... I was a bit yellow and very pale and in the evening I was really happy to have all of the anti-nausea drugs but apart from that, I ate lunch and dinner just fine, watched an episode of "Dr. Who" and slept very well.

On Thursday we went to get me unhooked from the IV and apart from feeling tired I was fine.

Then mid day on Thursday my aunt called and said that I should be nicer to my mom. I asked her why since I have been good and calling her several times a day. She said, well you know, they are a bit cooped up... Cooped up where?-I foolishly inquired... Well, in a hotel - my aunt said sheepishly... HOTEL WHERE? - I was getting a bit upset by this time... Well, somewhere in Houston - my aunt answered even more sheepishly... FOR HOW LONG???!... Since Tuesday...

Any way we have apparently been stalked for several days by two crazy Russian women... After talking with Richard and calming him down and realizing that they do have tickets home and do leave on Saturday, they were allowed into our house. They made us dinner and played with George and overall were not too much of a pain... YET... still have 2 days to go...

So where ever you are, and whatever you are doing, WATCH OUT for two crazy Russians... They may be following YOU....

Chapter 2
February 21, 2008

Well... It is about time of the week when I provide an update on my pro/regress...

You know how when you are a child your parents always tell you that you should be thorough in everything you do and do it properly once and for all? Well... So when the doctors and nurses told me that my white blood cells count is going to crash a week after the chemo, I did it properly, thoroughly reducing my count to more then ten times lower then expected. In other words even healthy people were too buggy for me. So when I went for my blood test on Wednesday I was already spiking fever and descending into the la-la land of delirium.

The natural reflex of the doctors and nurses in a situation like this is to fill you to the brim with antibiotics. So the nurse takes me to the room holding in her hand two humongous syringes full of some nasty antibiotic. The amount was so big that they had to give it to me in two doses, one in each hip. I did try my best to reason with the nurse and explain to her that even though I do have large hips there is no need to use an elephant - size syringe and the simple pediatric one will do. But deft to my pleas, she told me to lean against the observation table, pull my pants down and relax... so I asked her, in that case, to tell me when I can start enjoying myself as well... I think she thinks I am nuts...

I came home after the visit, ate lunch, and shook literally for 3 hours... I was freezing cold under 2 blankets with woolen socks and every muscle in my body ached. I now have a new appreciation of the meaning of the word "discomfort". I do not think I want to repeat the experience... By about 5pm I managed to warm up... By 10pm my fever broke... By 10:01 I started joking again... I guess some people just never learn!

Meanwhile, poor Richard was battling with George in the evening. George was in rather unco-operating mood yesterday and spent all evening "communicating" on the top of the lungs... just one sound over-and-over-and-over-and-over... So every time I surfaced from whatever new la-la show I was watching at a time, all I could hear was "AAAAAAH!!!!!!!!!!!!! AAAAAAAAAAH!!!!!!!!!!!! AAAAAAAAAAAAAH!!!!!!!!!!" The funny thing was he wasn't crying - just communicating... I think next time I'll ask for different soundtrack... something quieter and calming...a bit more music and a bit less screaming...

Chapter 3: Bye-bye hair
February 27, 2008

Thank you very much for tuning in to this broadcast. The management of this broadcast, of course, does not recognize that there are whole loads of more interesting and exciting things you rather be doing right now. Therefore, the length of this e-mail is kept as long as the management wishes.

Legal disclaimer: this chapter was written under the influence of a cocktail of very heavy drugs and another cocktail of drugs to counteract the side effects of the first cocktail. Because drug cocktails are like chips - you cannot have just one.

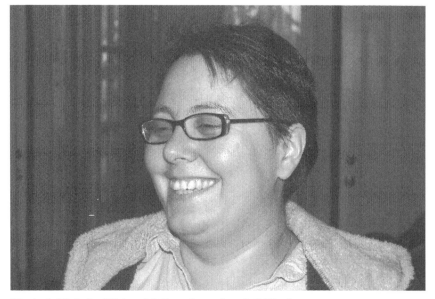

Photo 1. Hair by Richard "the scissor-hands" Clarke

On Wednesday I got a hair cut... This was soooo exciting!! More so, since Richard is the one who cut my hair in about 3 minutes before we had to rush off to the second cycle of chemo. If you talk with him any time soon, make sure to mention that you heard about his spiffing haircutting abilities. OK, so what that it is a bit crooked... or that I still have some long hair here and there... or that my bangs looks like something out of the horror movie... or that I, most likely, won't be allowed into children places so not to give them nightmares - who wants to go there anyway?... But he really did his best considering the face and the head he had to work with! I am even thinking of forgoing the trips to my expensive hair salon in the future and just letting him loose with scissors. And with all the money we can save on my hairdos we can buy him one expensive pair of scissors...

But let's go back to Monday… that was the day my hair showed the first signs of mutiny. It was first a trickle - a hair here and a hair there… But then they unionized… and when the negotiation with the hair union collapsed on Tuesday, it turned into flood. And I mean I **really** tried to compromise! First, on their demand, I stopped using hair dryers (in case they just flow away), then I had to wear a hat outdoors ("gone-with-the-wind" hairdo was not an option), no harsh chemicals (had to decide against dyeing them in bright red on that ground), loads of nutrient-rich conditioner.. I mean, how much else can one hair ask for?!! But they were still not happy. They were demanding a vacation! A VACATION!!! So I just had to put my foot down… and… well some of them are on vacation now… probably enjoying Cancun or wherever else nice the drainpipe will take them.. Others are packing as we speak... They did say there were no hard feelings and promised to send me a card… I am thinking of hiring new hair, but I was told that recruitment process might take several months...

I must here say something about my dear husband. Richard is very supportive through all this trying bad hair time. Once we were driving past a community sign wishing someone a Happy Birthday… I mentioned how nice it would have been if they were wishing me a happy birthday on that sign... So Richard looked at me, very supportively, and asked tenderly " So what do you want them to put there, honey: Happy Birthday, Baldy?" It really made me feel warm inside: not very many people are lucky enough to have such a caring and supporting husband like mine. Or there was that occasion when Richard, very happy for my achievements, mused over the fact that who would have thought that I am going to lose my hair before he loses his… It really made me feel proud that he is so happy for me… After all, every little thing counts (and gets remembered and recorded!)…

On the family front, George has decided that it is a prime time for him to be heard… and rather loudly… So when evil parents don't let him play with their computers or do other things he really want to do at that moment he takes a big breath, turns bright purple and

9

screams on top of his lungs (he also wiggles a lot and kicks if you happen to be holding him at that moment)… He is so hilarious and cute with his curly hair and huge drama crocodile tears and trembling lower lip that Richard and I are having such a laugh every time he does it! But, the "G. Clarkoshvili comedy shows" might be getting a bit more rare... Can it be that he actually doesn't want to be a stand up (actually sit down) comedian? Hm… need to ask him next time I see him… do not want to get him pigeon holed in a career he doesn't like at this early age…

Chapter 4: The rise of the shining head
March 5, 2008

I think that the biggest side effect of the chemo so far is that I am developing aversion to Wednesdays. Today is the Wednesday of the steroid crash, in a week is the Wednesday of chemo…

So today I have a steroid crash and feel like I have gotten a beating… then I have no feeling at the tips of my fingers (side-effect of one of the drugs)… then my eyes cannot focus well (side-effect of another drug)… then I have a sore throat - which is actually sores in my throat and a sore throat (side-effect of the whole shebang)... and then every time I sneeze, I have to run to the bathroom (God knows what caused this one!).. On top of it, my white blood cell count is even worse then 2 weeks ago…

But as the doctor told me today that if, with such a low blood count, the patient can answer "ok" on the question "how are you?", then it is simply a marvelous day!! Which put it all in a new perspective: apparently I am having a good day! So, all in all, I decided that today is a good day to write the next chapter!

Let start with last Friday when I had only a bald patch... on Saturday I had a comb-over... on Sunday I looked like badly plucked chicken… So … RICHARD SHAVED MY HEAD... Now my happy smiling face looks even more round and is quite dazzling if I do not wear a hat... It also gets a bit chilly to open the fridge or seat under A/C.

Now, how many of you men can boast that you have shaved your wife's head and LIVED to tell the tale? Ah? And all along the shaving (and that took about an hour to achieve a smooth shave) I could hear this quiet whispering ... faster and faster: "I am just a pleasant pheasant plucker, I much rather be pleasantly plucking pheasants"...

Then on Monday, just as I was getting acquainted with my new dazzling and shining look, a friend tried to sneak up to our house and deposit a pamelo (oriental grapefruit) at our door step. Now imagine my surprise when I looked in the bag and saw something

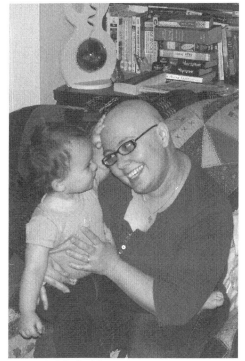

that looked just like my head! It was smooth and shiny with big cheeks and the right size too! At first I was contemplating preserving it for posterity, but then who wants to see a moldy version of his/her head? So I cut it... I was even more amazed when I found that inside of the pamelo was mostly padding... I must admit, it did put me into rather philosophical mood... Pamelo was quite tasty though... Since I am not supposed to eat acidic food and could only try a little piece, Richard is still eating it... stoically...

Photo 2. My bald head.

So I am wearing a turban now to prevent head freeze... You probably do not know that there were elections in Texas on

Tuesday. I am ashamed to tell that I have not gone to vote... I just imagined myself in a turban and with a mask and wearing gloves trying to convince the nice old ladies at the polling station that I am not a terrorist... I must admit I chickened out... But I reckon I can always make my voice heard the next time...

George has befriended my bald head...

Chapter 5: Descent of the BIG mama
March 12, 2008

It was nice and cool winter day in mid December of 2001. We were young and in Paris. After spending a day walking we were happy and tired. In the evening Richard took me in his loving arms, looked deep into my eyes with his beautiful dark eyes and asked me a question that redefined the rest of our lives: "Honey, can you promise that your mother will never Ever EVER live with us?"

You think I am kidding? Ask him! He only proposed AFTER I have reassured him that I am not THAT crazy. And I only agreed because he showed such wisdom at such a young age...

Now, since last Saturday, we are discussing whether 3 weeks living in the same house constitutes "living with us" and therefore is a breech of out prenuptial agreement... And all this because on Saturday afternoon my mama has descended on us to help...

My mama has a very different idea about what "help" means to most of the rest of us... It all started on bright Sunday mid-morning when she casually mentioned that there is a "little" problem with our bathroom upstairs. After Richard (still calmly) enquired whether she managed to block the toilet AGAIN, she replied indignantly that our toilet is just fine... but she had to take a shower knee-high in cold water. Showing first signs of worry, Richard foolishly asked why... "Because your bathtub doesn't drain water"... "What do you mean it DOESN'T drain water? IT WORKED FINE LAST NIGHT!"... "Well I do not know about last night, but my foots were cold while I take shower!" ... At this point Richard's nerves gave way under strain, so yelling "If she has pooped in the bathtub and blocked it, I WILL kill her" he rushed upstairs to investigate...

Now for some unknown reason my mama has this interesting effect on Richard: instead of his usual calm analytical self he becomes something very similar to a chicken running without its head. So he said "No worry... you just blocked it (please-please-please)... I am going to pour some nasty chemicals in the bathtub and it is going to (magically) unblock it". Deft to my pleas of postponing the procedure while we thoroughly assess the situation, he added a whole big jar of chemicals to the water... George's little rubber octopus was the first victim... My ears were the second (though I did learn a lot of new curse words in many languages)... Bathtub showed no signs or remorse...

After I talked Richard out of buying a gun and convinced him that we are too late to plant tomatoes this year anyway, we realized what my mama actually did. You know some bathtubs have this little lever that controls the built-in water stopper? Well not only she closed the drain, but she managed to break off the lever on the inside of the bathtub. So after a trip to the home improvement store, McGivering something out of coat hanger to keep the drain permanently open and mattering something about not trusting "that crazy woman"

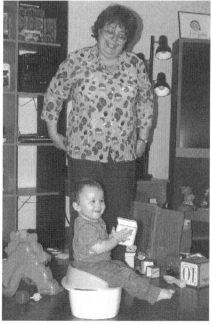

Photo 3. George and the queen of potties

with anything ever again, Richard has sealed the drain control forever. So, all in all, on Sunday evening we were much more exhausted than when we didn't have someone to "help" us.

I must give my mama a credit though. She did keep herself out of Richard's way after the "little incident" and is keeping George entertained. As a result he is now a proud possessor of THREE potties. I think mama thinks that there is a critical mass of potties after which George will finally get the idea. Well, if there is such a thing as potties critical mass then it is more than three! Overall though, she was so good that I was beginning to worry that the bathtub adventure would be the only thing I'll write about. Well she has fixed it today!

This Wednesday everything started as usual... until they could not get my port (built-in permanent IV access) to work for chemo. They stuck in a needle... then they moved it around... then they moved it some more... and some more... then they had to go and attend to my mother, who was trying to faint in a corridor... then they moved the needle some more... by this time mama was throwing up in the restroom... then they moved the needle some more... now mama was back with a very greenish tint to her face... then they moved the needle some more... then they forcefully sent mama to the waiting room with an order not to come back until she is called... then they changed the needle and finally got my port to work... then I calmly enquired whether they can give me something against a very unusual side effect of chemo I am having and the immediate reply was the "No, we cannot do anything about your mother!" ...

So... we are back to a gun and a tomato patch...

Chapter 6: The genius in each of us
March 19, 2008

Some of you told me last week to look at the positive side of mama's visit - the usual discomfort of Wednesday will not feel as bad in comparison.

And they were right!

Although I still lost most of the feeling in my fingers, cannot focus my eyes and have muscle ache all over my body, mama managed to keep me in good fighting spirit all day. You should see the grass next to our driveway! "What grass?" you would ask... EXACTLY! There is no more grass just very deep tire impressions... AND I WAS IN THE CAR WHILE SHE WAS DOING IT!!! Now, I may understand aversion to grass in someone who lives in Arizona, but what does she have against our neighbor's trees???

But let's pick up our story where we left off last time. Last Wednesday evening after the chemo I had an acute almost tearful nostalgia for my childhood. Mama made us a soup. It was just like I remembered: boiled whole chicken breast, boiled whole onion, boiled humongous matzo balls and no salt. After my valiant attempt at soup rescue spectacularly failed, mama reminded me that she has actually never claimed that she can cook. Damn right! However, this whole soup incident has put her in a mood of reminiscence about our childhood.

As most of you know, I have three brothers. The oldest was a child genius. According to mama, Igor could recite Pushkin and Shakespeare by the age of 1, count backwards and forwards by the age of 2, and most likely knew how to solve partial differential equations by the age of 3 only nobody thought to check. He was also a very kind and gentle boy until the age of about 1 and 3/4 at which point he started his scientific research on a topic of which toy is better to use for breaking Lena's head. (I did put an order for a new head when I got a bit older but I think it must have gotten lost in the mail)

After almost a week of listening about various childhood achievements of my older brother, Richard finally asked how come he has not heard anything about his wife's achievements yet. After initial sentiment of "well she was a girl and, you know, well...", mama gave us couple of hours of peace in which time she was frantically trying to figure out the nature of my genius... Finally, with great pride, she announced that she realized what was my inner genius... I COULD EAT!!! Apparently I could eat a lot, independently and with feeling from a very young age... "You should have seen her with a spoon!" proudly beamed mama at us...

But that was not it. Now since two of her kids were pure geniuses, what about the other two? With the slogan of "inside each child there is a genius" mama rushed to find the inner genius of my younger brothers... At last she found it!! YAN COULD POOP ("You should have seen him with the potty!") and BORIS COULD HIDE ("You should have tried to find him!").

And that leaves us with George... In the last couple of days mama is trying to find George's genius. Unfortunately, he neither speaks yet as his genius uncle Igor (although he communicates perfectly with grunts), nor does he handle the spoon as his genius mother (although the boy can eat!), nor has he figured out the inner working of the potty as his genius uncle Yanipoo (even with three potties surrounding him at all times), nor is he inclined to hide himself as his uncle Borihoodiny.. And to top it all, while his misunderstood genius, British uncle Gavywavy could draw as soon as he could hold a pencil, George simply eats crayons...

But I am not worried... we still have a week and a half before mama leaves... I am sure by that time we will definitely meet George's inner genius...

That leaves us with a question: what is Richard's inner genius? Or better yet... what is yours?

Chapter 7: The writer's block

March 26, 2008

Well, today I am going to simply update you on my progress - after all this is what these e-mails are all about, right?

My doctor said that she cannot feel any lumps under my skin any more - which I consider good news - the less extra lumps I have the better. I am going to have a second PET/CT on Friday to see how my internal lump is doing. I hope it is not doing well and, in fact, that it is completely gone. I also have to see a radiologist sometime soon in case the lump is still there and I need to radiate it.

I must admit I am not looking forward to being radiated but considering the alternative I will clench my teeth and take it like a man... hm... since sex change it not part of my treatment, lets try it again... I will clench my teeth and take it like a woman... hm... that doesn't sound all too good either, although true from a lot of different perspectives... how about this version... I will clench my teeth and take it like a human - complaining bitterly... Does anyone else feel sometime that the only reason we developed language was so we can complain?

Other than that, they had to scale down one of the drugs since my fingers are not doing too well. I kept burning and freezing them during the last two weeks. Usually, the type of chemo I am getting is administered every 3 weeks, but because I am strong and tough (and young) I am getting mine every 2 weeks. It's called "densed-in" schedule and has slightly better results then the usual 3 week schedule. That means that my nerves have one less week to recover between treatments. And, while they have a drug to counteract the white cell crash and bring it back up fast (although the doctor has been saying that she is impressed with my bone marrow ability to regenerate), I am on my own with my nerves. You know how surprised you get when you start feeling freezing pain in the middle of your finger that is not touching anything cold just to discover that you have a piece of frozen meet stuck to the top of it and you have not noticed! Well, if it doesn't get better until next time, the doctor was suggesting I get one week vacation from chemo… will see, I must admit I kinda want the chemo to be over soon - but I also want to still have my fingers when I am done… hair was optional. Especially since Richard has been "dead chuffed" that he has the most hair in the family at the moment. He is gloating now, but we'll see who has the last laugh!

And that brings us to the topic of writer's block. The last couple of days I have been thinking about what funny things happened to us during the last week so I can write to you about them. Unfortunately Richard and I are getting so used to living in the mad house, that the plumbing in the middle of the breakfast does not seem worthy of writing about anymore. So, yesterday, feeling under pressure from impeding chapter, I asked the family to suggest the topics.

I had a list of George's emerging inner geniuses that I collected from listening to mama, including but not limited to genius sleeper, genius eater and genius generalissimus (those of you who are not so intimately familiar with Russian history, please refer to the picture on the left)

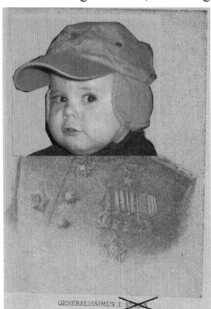

Photo 4. Generalissimus George

Richard suggested that the chapter should only have one line "Richard has been digging in the back yard all week-end". Which is true, but it is also true that after 2 hours of digging (Boy Scout motto: be prepared) he concluded that it is easier to send mama back to Arizona than digging a hole that is big enough for her…

18

Mama said that I should write about anything I want but her... Which surprised me a bit considering that I have been writing nothing but the truth about her...

George said "Eeeehhhh!"

So after careful consideration of all of the suggestions, here it is:

Eeeehhhh!

Chapter 8: In the eye of the storm
April 2, 2008

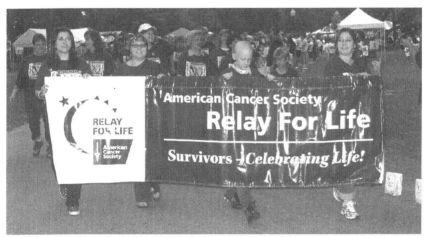

Photo 5. The banner girl

Let me start this chapter with the words that we are so used to by now: it is Wednesday and I feel like crap. However, due to a preemptive antibiotic treatment that I started on Monday and smaller dose of one of the chemo drugs, I feel like one of the better smelling varieties. But as always, my eyes don't focus, my fingers don't feel and my muscles ache. Other than that, everything is absolutely spiffing. And because we have established my blood count pattern, I don't even have to give blood today. So life is definitely looking up!

Last Friday THE FAMILY participated in a fundraising walk for the American Cancer Society. With help from our friends and family we raised more than $4300! However, while most of the people were honoring those lost to cancer and celebrating life, Richard was celebrating survival: mama has been with us for 3 weeks. He had to survive for only another 2 days! Needless to say, for the last 3 days he was positively beaming and in the best mood ever. I, on the other hand, have been worrying that with mama gone home, our life will become boring and I will have nothing to write to you about.

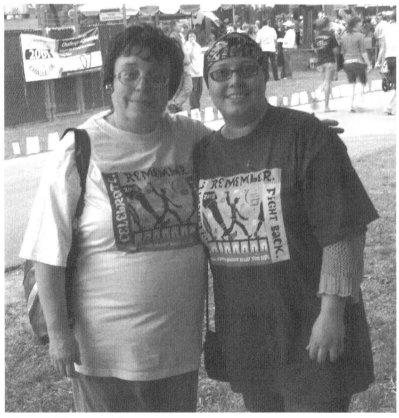

Photo 6. Mama and I

You see, this Friday my mother-in-law is coming to stay with us for almost a month. However, compared to my mom, who is intensely "unique" and behaves in "extraordinary" ways, Richard's mom is pleasantly eccentric.

However, last Sunday, as if to alleviate my worry, my mother-in-law has been attacked by a compost heap in her back yard and apparently now looks like a football hooligan after a bar brawl. So if I now get "LOVE" and "HATE" tattoos on my shining head, my mother-in-law and I will look like a perfect couple out of bikers paradise. But all of this means that on Friday instead of having to take care of an invalid and a baby, Richard will have to take care of TWO invalids and a baby.

That, together with my father trying to cure an infection from a cactus thorn by means of poison ivy (apparently poison ivy works better than antibiotics - perhaps I should try it one of these Wednesdays) and getting lost in the bottom of a canyon knee-high in cold water, makes me think that it is never going to be boring in our household.

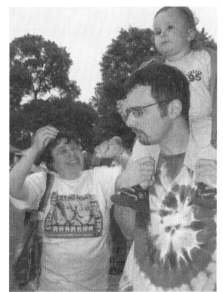

**Photo 7. Only 2 more days!
I WILL SURVIVE!!!**

Chapter 9: Bye-bye cancer!
April 10, 2008

Apologies to the dear audience for being a bit late with this chapter, but as people who went through same chemo before predicted, after chemo #4 it gets a bit tougher, so I was flat on my back for 2 days trying to get enough energy back for typing.

Aside from all of that, a great event occurred yesterday: I finally had a proof of how remarkably observant my husband is. Right before we left for chemo, Richard looked at me thoughtfully and, a MONTH AND A HALF after I started to wear scarves ALMOST EVERY DAY, asked me whether I am matching my scarf color to my clothes (which I have always done from day one). As I said before, with every day I get more and more proof that I could not have chosen a husband with keener awareness of his surroundings.

And another miracle happened today. I have been driven to the doctor's office by my British mother-in-law who only drove in Houston once before. I am proud to announce that I have not screamed, neither have I attempted to grab the wheel, nor have I put my scarf over my eyes and whimpered. Overall it was a rather peaceful journey but we did have to calm our nerves with a nice medicinal chocolate mousse after we got home.

Another great achievement came on George's front: we finally managed to catch his #1 into the potty. Now all we need to do is catch his #2 and make him communicate to us when his majesty desires to get on the potty. That said, we received a perfect explanation of why George is having difficulty with potty training from our good friend Steve. He thinks that George is just very good in math and thinks along the following lines that make perfect sense: "Why three potties? Sure, three is a nice little prime number, but so is two. Well, one plus two is three, so maybe I am supposed to use potty three when I need to do both? But what if I'm on one doing one, and get the urge to do two? Do I stop and go to potty three or finish and go to potty two? It's so confusing. I sure hope they don't bring home a fourth potty!"

Apart from that, everything has been relatively peaceful on the home front thanks to the preemptive placement of a plunger next to my mother-in-law's toilet, although the side effects of my mother's visit are still felt. Right before mama left, she proclaimed that we are not eating enough sour cream and cabbage, bought us both, and drove to the airport to catch a flight to Tucson. Now what do you do with a large tub of sour cream and a huge amount of cabbage if you really not into both of those things? You use weird recipes and improvise! So we ended up with a la Russian cabbage cake. It was actually not bad but there was quite a lot of it. So we ate it stoically for Sunday lunch. We aired the house. We ate it even more stoically for dinner. But by breakfast time I had a full blown revolt on my hands. After a long negotiation we finished the cake on Tuesday, but I do not think we will be eating cabbage again any time soon… But if you ask me, the cabbage cake was one of the nicest things I could have made them eat!

And now, here is something you have probably been waiting for: the results of my PET/CT scan. I am proud to announce that according to the radiologist who did the reading of the results I had an "excellent chemotherapeutic response". **No lymphoma could be identified on the scan**. And that means that I have no lesions measuring 5mm or more. So we have survived the cancer! Now I just need to survive the rest of the treatment. No matter how much I begged and whined the doctor was pretty determined on me finishing my last 2 chemo treatments (I have only one left now) and she strongly recommended that I follow that up with a month of radiation therapy since my cancer was pretty aggressive and we do not want to leave a cell of two behind that will divide into new lumps later. On the bright side, no matter what the side effects of radiation are, the side effects of more chemo are much worse. So in mid-May I will start daily radiation therapy and we will have this chapter of my life behind us by mid June.

I must admit I didn't know how worried I was about getting better until I learned the results of the test. Suddenly my life even with my senseless and periodically infecting fingers, bad Wednesdays and overall tiredness looks much more cheerful!

Chapter 10: And life's your lobster

April 16, 2008

When we first got the house, Richard and I used to spend a lot of time gardening. But with George and all, our back yard has gotten in a rather more natural state of mind. And when I say natural, I mean bushes taller than our garage roof, opossums and raccoons, and house plants nesting up the trees and mutating into blood-thirsty monsters with leaves at least a foot in diameter. So when Richard suggested to Dorne (my mother in law) that, if she is bored, she can do some gardening, my biggest concern was that she was going to be eaten by something lurking at the back of the garden. But apparently I have underestimated her. Armed with a crowbar and a pair of rather large snip-snips, she has successfully cleared up our back yard of most of the plants. No, I really mean it! Instead of bushes we now have quite short leafless trunks, the mutant plant is gone and so are most of the other "useless" little trees. But we now have 24 cucumber plants on a patio and we might even have some tomato plants later. We are also discovering the marvels of upside-down gardening.

Do you know that, allegedly, you can grow plants upside-down? Well, allegedly, you can and, allegedly, it works well for plants like tomato, cucumber and other vines. You can either buy a special planter for lots of money or … you can make your own! Needless to say that buying planters is for wimps, so armed with an empty tetra pack milk carton, my old nylon sock, a glue gun and a bit of rope, we made an upside-sown planter, stuck a poor-little-sod-of-a-flower in it and hung it off a branch of one of the few remaining trees in our back-yard. Looks absolutely awful but so far works! So all we need is 24 plastic soda bottles and 24 old nylon socks (Note from Richard: NO! This is NOT a request for you to donate your dirty old socks. I do NOT want to find old socks on my desk when I arrive at work in the morning!) and our cucumber plantation will be well on its way! That will teach Richard to go on a business trip leaving me and his mom alone!!

Apart from upside-down gardening, I was also teaching Dorne to drive an automatic car. Since today is my bad day and I cannot see well, Dorne volunteered to drive to pick George up from the nanny. Only she wanted a practice drive around the neighborhood first, since she had never driven an automatic car before. Now you would think that, with the car being automatic, there is nothing to teach. Well I thought so too!

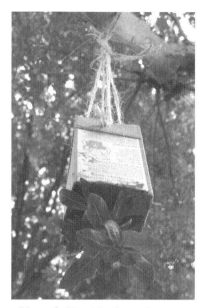

Photo 8. Up-side-down flower

So, Dorne gets in the driver seat, I get into the passenger seat, she adjusts the mirrors, I buckle up, she turns the key, I tell her how to put the car in gear... the stick would not move. Yelling "I have not done anything! It is not my fault! I have not even touched anything yet because you told me not to!" Dorne tries to move the stick up, she tries to move the stick down, I try to move it up and down, she tries to move the stick right and left, I try to move it right and left - the stick would not bulge! "No worries!" said I beginning to worry. With a hypothesis that it is just some kind of anti-theft-by-mother-in-law-security-thing, we got out of the car, locked the doors, unlocked the doors, I got on the driver's seat, turn the car on, washed the windshield for good measure and... moved the stick into gear! With "all fixed, now you try!", I turned off the car, got out, Dorne got into the drivers side, turned on the car, attempted to put the car in gear... the stick would not move... By that time I was getting a pretty strong feeling that my car is trying to warn me about something important; Dorne was crying with laughter. Finally, after about the fifth attempt, Dorne was proudly sitting in the driving seat with the car on and in gear.

Do you know how disconcerting it is to find oneself looking at your mother in law grinning from ear to ear through the windshield of a car at you? Especially realizing that you are on the other side? And that you actually have no idea whether the car is in drive or reverse or, for that matter, whether your mother in law is aware that she is supposed to be pressing the brake continuously? Well... After a couple of uncomfortable moments, we were both in the car and with lots of noises of delight at no need to shift gears and a bit of a confusion over a spare foot that wanted to be put somewhere, we finally proceeded to have our practice drive and rode off into the sunset... actually more like Houston smog.

Chapter 11: The chemo brains
April 25, 2008

On Monday I went for lunch with a friend of mine and complained to her that my short term memory and especially the ability of looking up correct words is somewhat sluggish. So, I was musing the fact that my brain cells are being wiped out by chemo... We laughed about it... But the next day I read in the headline news from the BBC about a phenomenon that is called "chemo brains". Essentially it is the coating on the neurons that is fast dividing and has to be renewed constantly and if it doesn't the connections go bust, brains shrink and turn into pumpkin...

So being somewhat worried I (foolishly as usual) decided to look for support from my dear hubby... So he turns to his mom and says: "You know, mom, when I married her she even had brains!" After a short period of domestic violence, he added in effort to calm me down: "Don't worry about your brains, honey! You know that I married you for your looks... your beautiful sparkly eyes, your cheerful smile, and your wonderful wavy brown hair... uhh... hmmm... well they should come back soon, right?"

Seeing as Richard was heading toward the imminent meat grinder, Dorne, being a constant optimist, suggested a completely different attitude to the whole brains/short memory problem. She said that I now have a perfect excuse forever... "Honey you wanted that dinner an hour ago? Oops sorry, completely forgot: chemo brain"... or ... "You mean you wanted me to help you to clean up? Oops, sorry completely forgot: chemo brain!" ... or... "You mean you didn't want me to spend all that money on shopping? Oops sorry: chemo brain!"... Or even better... "Bill/Matt, you mean I was supposed to work on that horribly boring project? Oops sorry, completely forgot - chemo brain!"

Well, somewhat cheered up by all of the excuses I can now use, I decided to talk with my doctor and see if she thinks that chemo-brain is real. So on Wednesday before my LAST chemo, I casually enquire whether she thinks that my brains are being affected. The answer was short and clear "Yep"... hmm... When I asked whether there is anything I can do about it, the answer was even clearer "Nope"... She did say, however, that it will get better in the future and that all of the side-effects should disappear with time... But for now, if there anything I was supposed to do and didn't (or didn't want to): "Sorry, I have a chemo brain!

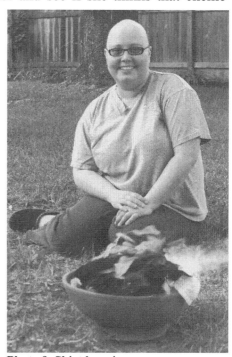

Photo 9. Shirt burning ceremony

Did I mention that it was my LAST chemo?! Well it was! I even got a graduation certificate from the nurses: something about courage and persistence, good spirit and generally being a pain-in-the-butt. So, to celebrate the occasion, today we had a ceremony of

27

burning of my chemo shirts. Because, believe me, there is absolutely no way I am going to want to wear them again!

Chapter 12: The brave new world
April 30, 2008

Hurray! I have a steroid crash and what a wonderful occasion it is!

No! No! It is not an affect of my chemo brain: the reason for celebration is absolutely genuine. Today is the last chemo related steroid crash - the final kick in my chemo saga. The chemo part of my life is now slowly slipping into the realm of legends. Also, my mother-in-law is going home today, so starting this evening we are assumed to be capable of taking care of ourselves on our own (God help us!). Here is the final tally of planting impacts of my mother-in-law on the Clarkoshvili crazy farm:

14 upside-down planters; 24 cucumber plants; 97 tomato plants; countless marigolds, sunflowers and, possibly, chives; 1 pepper plant; 1 eggplant; 1 rosemary bush; 3 strawberry plants; 4 blackberry bushes; 1.5 dewberry bushes; 1 rehabilitated plumbago plant; 1 rehabilitated jasmine plant; Cherry pot experiment with at least 20 pips from dried sour cherries; Yellow pepper experiment with countless seeds from store bought pepper; melon experiment with countless seeds from store bought melon; dill experiment with countless several-year-old dill seeds from my mom's garden

On the wish list for next season is the medicinal marijuana. (We couldn't find any seeds in the local nursery this year).

And last but not least - George's college fund: thousands of dug-up Nerine bulbs - 2/$7 in the neighborhood nursery and on-line. Beautiful in bloom and nutritious, our local daredevil, Chinese geophysicist-chef serves them up in an exotic, gourmet cuisine that will bring color to your kitchen and tears to your eyes! We offer discount prices! Sign up while supplies last!

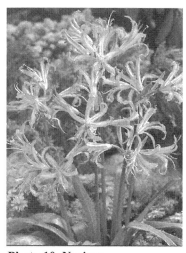
Photo 10. Nerines

But yes, my dear friends, the chemo saga has come to an end and next week I will enter the brave new world of going to work, radiation and growing hair. I promise to keep you updated with the rest of my treatment and going-ons on the our crazy farm, but it will not be as regular as before. So thank you very much for your kind thoughts and wishes and patience with my delirious writing!

Until the next update!

Chapter 13: One year after
March 20, 2009

Ooph... It has been only a year since I wrote the first chapter of my saga but it seems like a long-long-long-long time ago. After the chemo was over, I got scanned and measured for a face mask and harness to keep me in place during radiation therapy. They also drew three marks on my front and two on my sides in bright purple permanent ink so that they could align me within millimeters of the position I had during the original scan. Deft to my pleas, they refused to draw a smiley face between my color bones but agreed to draw a smile on my mask. Man, it looked spooky! The radiologist promised me that after 2 weeks of radiation I will, FINALLY, start losing weight. After the third week we concluded that it takes much more than a little suntan on my esophagus for me to lose my appetite. Eating, after all, is my inner genius! After I asked for my money back, I got to keep my mask... A sort of short and voluptuous Hannibal Lector...

I did, however, start losing weight out of the blue a couple of weeks AFTER the radiation, which almost drove me into a panic -

that had been the first sign of my cancer before. But we have since decided that it must have been taking lots of energy to grow my new crop of hair. After regular watering, weeding and fertilizing, I had an inch-long, very thick and curly hair-cover by September. They were, unfortunately, almost all white, a feature that has remarkably disappeared since (yeah!!!) together with curls and thickness (sigh...). What did drive me into a complete panic was discovering a large lump in the top middle of my abdomen one night in August. With a torrential downpour of tears and earthquake-force sobs I woke Richard up. As usual, reveled by an opportunity to show me some more support, and with "Congratulations, honey! You have FINALLY discovered your chest bone!", he rolled to the other side and fell asleep again. The presence of my chest bone was confirmed by my oncologist, gynecologist (he got lost), PET scan and, most important of all, the internet. Since that time, I try to socialize with my lymph nodes on a regular basis in case they start multiplying out of boredom. It must be working - so far, no more lumps.

To add to the excitement, hurricane Ike visited in early September. Our house was mostly undamaged but we were without power for a week. We woke up to a peacefully quiet house. The phones were dead... the A/C was off... Our fridge was packed with food conspiring to go off... by the time we contacted mama at 7am her time, she was already packing my grandmother into a car ready to drive off to Houston (Yeah! Like that would have helped!). After giving us a long stream of mutually contradicting motherly advice, and with: "If you do not have power and A/C, AT LEAST TURN ON YOUR CEILING FANS!" she indignantly hung up. Completely bedazzled, Richard turned on the switch for the ceiling fan as if by some magical power mama managed to get electricity into the circuit... Overall, Ike was a time of abundance of food (since everything in everybody's fridges had to be eaten fast), great sleep-overs at our friends (they had power) and relaxing time off work clearing up the mess in our backyard.

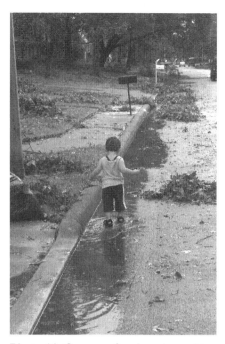

Photo 11. George after hurricane Ike

By mid-autumn mama's patience had worn out. After deciding that I had enough time in the spotlight, she had one of those mysterious "now you see it, now you don't" heart attacks. She was admitted to the hospital while allegedly having a heart attack and was dismissed by the end of the day with permission to go to work the next day when the next shift of doctors couldn't find any signs of any kind of present, past or future heart troubles. While mama was relaxing in the hospital bed, my gran was wailing encouragingly "my poor-poor daughter is going to die" by her side... the whole time (eight hours)… And the only thing mama did to set it off was to faint at the sight of a needle as usual! Thank God, they are both fine now!

In mid November, we had three "we made it" birthday celebrations. I made it to 34! After that I got in a rather thoughtful mood about my future retirement. Since people who have a hobby they love live longer and happier lives, Richard will be the happiest multicentarian in 2500s. I, on the other hand, do not have a clear idea of what to do when I retire. So, I thought of becoming a professional doodler in my old age. The idea was to have a little café in a tiny village in the South of France where I doodle while talking with customers who happily buy my doodles while chatting with me over coffee. But I don't fancy waking up early, working week-ends and never having a vacation, neither do I want to bake for a living, nor do I like to do dishes and clean… Oh yeah! And I do not speak French… Apart from these minor details, Richard pointed out with his usual quiet demeanor, it was quite a good idea!... Bummer!... So if you have any suggestions about my future potential hobby, I will be happy to consider them all.

George is now a boisterous 2-year-old who rules the nest. He started speaking in a way, but you will need a bi-lingual translator to understand him. Although, when it comes to demanding cakes, cookies, juice or balloons he is perfectly clear. A month ago he started attending Russian Saturday school where they actually SIT FOR 45 MINUTES for each lesson – a feat I would not believe possible if I wouldn't have seen it with my own eyes.

He started swimming lessons in September and for the first 3 month they were actually "screaming" lessons. We had our routine – come, see the pool, throw-up, get cleaned up, get in the pool and scream for the whole 30-min-long lesson. Although it is still a routine, since December it has been slightly modified – come, see the pool, attempt a head-first dive, get rescued by a parent, get in the pool, tell teacher off for doing stuff in the wrong order, scream when the lesson is over.

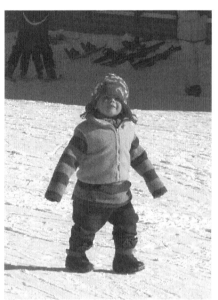

Photo 12. Our little snow gipsy

At Christmas we went to visit UK for a week, where George was really happy to see all of the sheep, cows, horses, wolves, tigers and bears. All within 10 minutes walk from his grandparents' house! After that we spent 2 weeks on top of the Pyrenees just when they were having record amount of snow. George did not really like the snow – it is cold and wet especially when one is refusing to wear mittens and keeps falling face first in it. So he was wearing all of his sleeves extra-long. He also didn't always like his snowsuits, so most of the time he resembled a coat hanger with haphazardly hanged clothes. Of course we all got sick and with remarkable precision of a doctor visit every 2-days befriended the French medical system. We spent a day in Paris on the way back. George really liked Paris with its trains and busses. If it was up to George... and me and Richard... we would have probably stayed there. Well, now we are back to normal routine, trying to get some rest before our trip to my mama in Arizona in a week's time.

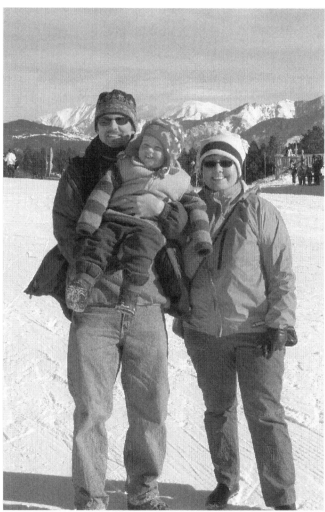

Photo 13. Clarkoshvilis in Pyrenees

Chapter 14: When to stop writing
Summer / Fall 2009

I sincerely apologize for the delay of getting the book out. I have no excuse apart from general laziness and slight annoyance at the fact that life is not as amusing as it was while I was on drugs. That said some things have not changed... Mama visited for a week in early summer and our shower immediately broke and started spewing water upward and over the curtain watering our ceiling and everything else in the bathroom apart from mama who was patiently waiting for water in the bathtub. Even after Richard fixed it, she ended up taking cold shower because having PhD in math doesn't quite prepare one for intricacies of operating hot/cold water controls. All that apart, Richard and I actually enjoyed her visit in early summer. We went to the cinema 3 times, which is 2 times more than in the first 2 years of George's life.

Shortly after mama left for Tucson, I got pecked by a bird on the top of my head. Now, how many of you can claim a similar achievement, ah? I think I must have a homing devise implanted in my... somewhere... and transmitting "me! me! pick me!". Especially since my coming to America was actually celebrated with NewYorkan seagull pooping on my head. Richard of course had a ball pouring alcohol on my head and explaining to George that it is ok to do this to mommy because she is "special".

George went through a phase when he decided that he doesn't want to be called by any nicknames anymore and his name is only George. So in order to teach him a lesson of "be careful what you ask for" we have been teaching him his full name. So far all we got is George Sososilly Clak and a full reversal on "no nick name" policy. His speech has progressed a lot from "What's that noise?" and "What's in there?" at 2½ to "What's that mean?" to "What's that smell? Pewee! Papa, go to potty!" at 2¾.

Yes, the slow and relaxing "terrible twos" are almost over and the brave new world of much faster and louder "terrifying threes" is knocking at our door... If life continues the way it is going now, the parents might not survive much longer... Did I mention that George took both of ours stubbornness and multiplied them together? Or that he took complete disregard for peer pressure from his father and for authority from his mother? And just to make it all more exciting, he also picked up some aptitude for completely crazy and mischievous ideas from his mother and devious mind to work them to perfection from his father! In other words, think not just twice but many times before having children - they are not what you think but exactly what people warn you about in horror movies!

Richard has finally showed who the man in the house is. While I was valiantly dueling with a humongous wasp in George's room without regard for my own safety and with only thought of my family's well being in mind, Richard was hiding behind my back squealing like a school girl. Of course, once the wasp was semi-dead, he emerged from the safety of my broad torso, finished off the wasp and took all the credit. But I forgave him! Don't mention it to him but when he was not right BEHIND me, Richard's underwear proved crucial in protecting my life from nasty flying cockroach. That pair of underwear will never be the same... No need to worry him...

There is also new development on the front of my last name. My very kind and attentive co-workers, while purely concerned and full of eagerness to ease the hardship of explaining how to pronounce my last name, came up with a way to teach it once and for all. Here it comes:

"Sh! Oh, shit! Ay!" shvili.

To top it off a friend of mine decided that "exuberant" is pretty much one word summary of my personality. Now you understand why I just have to go back for more drugs???

Chapter 15: The splashy ending

October 21, 2009

Well… I have sincerely hoped that my book was finished. I have even contacted an on-line publishing company! But, I guess, it didn't quite have splashy enough ending, so I went ahead and created it today. To paraphrase Richard, I live to please my audience!

As usual for this time of the year, last week I went to get my PET scan. I came, got injected with radioactive sugar, lost most of my vision and had one of the worst headaches of my life while being scanned. Coincidence? Sure!

In the week between the test and the result I had an acute case of stress shopping. I bought most of the clothes that George will need for the next two years (in case the test was bad) and new shoes for myself (in case the test was good). Seeing how the money was trickling out of our nest-egg, Richard tried to reassure me that if the test is bad, Georges clothes will be the least of his worries. Well, of course, that completely back fired! My shopping has only intensified as the images of George in Walmart clothes started to flash in front of my eyes.

So… Today the wait was over. Today was exciting! I went to get my semi-annual top-up on mind bending drugs. It was all going so well: all-clear PET scan, new shoes discussion with my doctor, blood test, jokes with the nurses… Then my nurse accessed my port with an IV line, "flushed" it with saline solution… and all hell broke loose…

My head felt funny and quite heavy, then the neck, then I lost 90% of my vision, then I couldn't feel my left arm, then my legs… Oh my God! I MUST BE HAVING A STROKE!!! Realizing that I am also having difficulties talking got me completely freaked out (me and talking – we are tight!). With a yelp "Hug me! I am scared! I am too young to die!" I latched onto the neck of my nurse, buried my face in her voluptuous and welcoming bosom and broke into uncontrollable whimpering.

Of course, everything described in the previous paragraph happened in about 5 milliseconds. For my nurse the events went

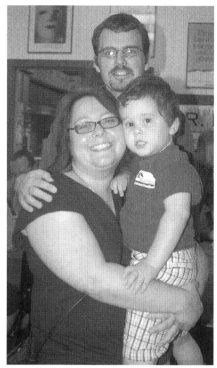
Photo 14. 35 and counting!

something like: she injected saline solution, she got hugged! Completely shocked by my outpouring of feelings and bewildered by my reaction to the saline solution ("For God's sake, woman! NOBODY dies from the saline solutions!"), my nurse checked my blood pressure (it was slightly elevated... surprise- surprise!) and called my doctor. The doctor arrived, looked, listened and concluded that I have developed a subconscious dislike of getting intravenous injections. In other word, my body freaks out and produces a vesicular spasm in my brain, hence the head-ache and the whole hoop-la-la.

Still... I was quite a star! Everyone in the office was around me trying to calm me down and offer their support to the poor nurse who was still being tightly hugged. Needless to say my nurse was not going to put anything else in me today in case I would express my affection for her even further. She disconnected me from IV, flushed my port ... I lost my vision ... This time, however, we were prepared and managed to avoid the exuberant bodily contact.

Now I have to go and see a neurologist and get my head screwed on right (if it is even possible). After all, it is quite unseemly to have a complete nervous break down every time at the sight of a needle. Oh my God! Somebody help me!! I am turning into my mama!!! Arhhh!!!!

And here is a philosophical dilemma: should I wait and tell you what the neurologist said or should I finish the book now? In spite of everything that was happening to me lately, let's hope that there will be something happening to me later at least for a while yet. So, nah, I think the book is as good now as it will ever be… in its as incomplete as my life state… And the future… well let's hope it will be too boring to deserve a separate book…

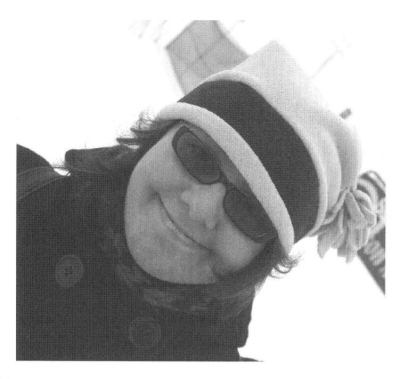

About the author:

Elena grew up in Moscow, Russia and moved to the US at the age of 20. After exciting 8 months in the Bronx, she moved to Tucson, Arizona and almost a decade later to Houston, Texas. Somewhere along the way in Tulsa, Oklahoma, Elena met Richard. (Where else?!).

Elena, Richard, their son George and their 2½ cats live in Houston, TX where they are entertaining themselves with perpetual remodeling of their house.

4789789R0

Made in the USA
Charleston, SC
17 March 2010